Sugar

7 Day Sugar Junkie Detox Diet Plan To Beat Your Addiction And Rescue Yourself From Cravings Easily And Naturally With Clean Eating Recipes For Life!

Sarah Brooks

STOP!!! Before you read any further....Would you like to know the Secrets of Body Transformation?

If your answer is yes, then you are not alone. Thousands of people are looking for the secret to rapidly burn body fat, keep the weight off, become healthier, and truly transform their body and life for good.

If you have been searching for these answers without much luck, you are in the right place!

Not only will you gain incredible insight in this book, but because I want to make sure to give you as much value as possible, right now for a limited time you can get full **100% FREE access to a VIP bonus EBook** entitled **THE 7 KEYS TO BODY TRANSFORMATION!**

Just Go Here For Free Instant Access:

www.liveFitVIP.com

Legal Notice

Disclaimer Notice

Table Of Contents

Introduction

I want to thank you and congratulate you for purchasing the book, "Sugar: 7 Day Sugar Junkie Detox Diet Plan To Beat Your Addiction And Rescue Yourself From Cravings Easily And Naturally With Clean Eating Recipes For Life!"

This "Sugar" book contains proven steps and strategies on how to cut down your sugar intake in seven days without compromising your health.

This book includes:

- Recipes that will help reduce your consumption of sugar and carbohydrates.
- A simple 7-day meal plan that will help lower down your sugar cravings and help you lose weight.
- Helpful tips on how to stick on this detox and reap its maximum benefits.

The recipes contained in this book are also ideal for diabetics who wish to detoxify their body and reverse their Diabetes.

Whether you are suffering from diabetes or you are simple addicted to sugar and wants to live a healthier life, this book can help you achieve the healthier version of you.

Start flipping those pages and learn how to get in shape effectively.

Thanks again for purchasing this book, I hope you enjoy it!

Chapter 1: What Is Sugar Addiction?

Sugar addiction is the dependence on sugar consumption. People who are addicted to sugar commonly eat more than they intend to, they crave for sugar and they lose control. Sugar addicts can't stop eating sweet treats such as cakes, pastries, soda and other carbohydrates-filled foods and products.

According to experts, eating sugar causes the brain to release more Dopamine, which is a neurotransmitter that plays a major role in a person's emotions, sense of pleasure and pain, drive and desire to get things done. When we eat sugary foods in large amounts, it causes the Dopamine receptors to downgrade. Therefore, there are fewer receptors for Dopamine. When this happens, the next time we consume foods that have high sugar content the effect is considerably weaker than before; which is why we need to eat more to get the same feeling.

Due to the effects of sugar to the rewards center of the brain, sugar addiction functions the same as drug abuse such as nicotine and cocaine. Just like drug addiction, people get addicted to sugar and lose control over their consumption. This is basically how sugar affects the brain so that we crave for more and eat more.

Sugar addiction can lead to a myriad of health issues such as heart diseases, binge eating, cravings and weight gain. Research also shows that a diet rich in sugar increases the risk for Type II Diabetes, causes significant decrease in HDL (good) cholesterol and elevated triglycerides. Too much sugar intake is also linked to migraine, depression, poor eyesight, gout, osteoporosis and autoimmune diseases such as multiple sclerosis and arthritis.

The more sugar we consume, the more tolerant we become. Our strong craving for sugar is not because of our genes. It is actually due to our food choices and dietary habits. This means you can reverse the effects of sugar addiction. Sugar Detox Diet is an effective way of cutting down on sugar consumption. Once you have undergone a Sugar Detox Diet, you will no longer have cravings for sweet treats and you will start eating better.

Chapter 2: Signs And Symptoms Of Sugar Addiction

Most of us have experienced cravings for sweet foods at one point in our lives. But how do you know if you are indeed suffering from sugar addiction.

Below are the clues that you may be addicted to sugar:

- You consistently crave for sugar or something sweet. For example, you crave for something sweet every morning, midday, afternoon or evening. This can be an indication that you have become dependent on sugar to appease your emotional downturns or jumpstart your energy on those specific times.

- You eat sweet, starchy or carbohydrates-filled foods even when you are not hungry. Due to cravings, you lose control over your eating habits. You eat sweet foods even of you are not hungry just to satisfy your cravings.

- You feel sleepy or tired after eating sugary foods. This happens because too much consumption of sugar causes a surge of insulin levels in your blood. When the insulin levels in your blood overcompensate, the brain signals the body to stop body functions. Therefore, you feel lethargic, tired or sleepy.

- You feel a great deal of discomfort when you try to control your sugar consumption. When you are not able to consume your usual sweet foods, you feel symptoms like headaches, nausea, moodiness, irritability and fatigue. This means your body is craving for more sugar, causing withdrawal symptoms.

- You tend to eat more and more of your favorite sweet foods to satisfy your cravings each day. Due to the reduction of dopamine receptors in your brain, your body requires more sugar to achieve the same level or satisfaction you experienced the last time.

Sugar is readily available in most of the foods we consume today. Sugar is in soda, fruit juices, ice cream, pastries, cakes, breads, cookies and other processed foods. It is no surprise obesity and Type II Diabetes is increasing. Our food choices affect our health and we can be in control if we choose to.

Chapter 3: Sugar And Its Negative Effects To The Body

In its basic definition, sugar (table sugar) is the combination of glucose and fructose, which are monosaccharides or simple sugars. Glucose is found naturally in fruits and vegetables. The human body also produces glucose naturally, but it does not produce fructose. If taken in very low amounts, the liver converts it into glycogen and stores it for future use. But, if taken excessively, the liver will be overloaded with glycogen. As a result, it forces the liver to convert the fructose into fats, which can lead to fatty liver, insulin resistance, diabetes, obesity and a myriad of other diseases.

Studies also show that fructose, which is found is sugar, decreases the level of nitric oxide in the body and raises angiotensin, leading to muscle contraction. When this happens, your blood pressure is raised, potentially causing damage to your liver.

Sugar is also the major cause of obesity. This substance does not fill you up. As a matter of fact, sugar tricks your body's metabolism by turning off the appetite-control system so that you gain more weight. Sugar does not properly stimulate insulin, therefore, it does not suppress the hunger hormone known as ghrelin and the satiety hormone (leptin) is not stimulated. This is why you eat more and you develop insulin resistance.

Experts also believe that increased consumption of sugar increases your risk of cancer. Cancer is the uncontrolled multiplication and growth of cells, an insulin regulates this kind of growth. Therefore, increased insulin levels can greatly contribute to the formation of cancer cells. Moreover, metabolic problems linked to sugar are drivers of inflammation, a possible cause of cancer.

Due to the effect of sugar to the Dopamine receptors in the brain, you feel sluggish and irritated afterwards. Furthermore, sugar has no nutrients and experts consider it as an empty calorie. Therefore, your hunger is not satiated. Instead, it makes you crave for more afterwards. This is why sugar addicts gain weight fast and their cravings are uncontrollable.

Chapter 4: Blood Sugar Solution

To reduce your risk of diabetes and insulin resistance, you must follow a blood sugar solution. To ensure optimal blood sugar balance in your blood, follow these simple guidelines:

Eat natural, unprocessed foods such as fruits and vegetables. Stay away from chemical-laced processed foods at all costs.

Eat low-glycemic carbohydrates in moderate amounts only.

While undergoing blood sugar therapy, you must avoid any foods containing gluten and all dairy products for your gut to heal effectively.

Follow and complete your blood solution program strictly for a successful outcome.

You need to eliminate all foods, drinks and habits that can cause a spike in your blood sugar levels. This means all types of grains, sugar, sweeteners, and starchy foods are taboo during your detox. Even legumes and beans are off limits. This is because carbohydrates-heavy foods, sugar and starches causes a spike in blood sugar. It is not easy for your body to digest beans and legumes, and they can cause stomach issues so you need to eliminate them during your detox. You may reintroduce them to your system slowly later on.

A blood sugar solution detox usually lasts up to 7 days. During this period, you can eat three well-balanced meals with healthy snacks in between. The idea is to flush out all the toxins in your body by strictly following a sugar-free, low-carb diet for 10 days. After the detox, you will no longer feel the craving for sweet foods, you will feel more alive and your symptoms such as bloating, migraine, headache, gas, etc. will be relieved.

You will soon realize that fruits and vegetables are better, compared to those sweet concoctions you used to gobble up. Your body will slowly go back to its natural state before the toxins corrupted your system. Due to this, you will experience withdrawal symptoms in the first 3 to 4 days of your detox. These symptoms include mood swings, nausea and intense craving for food. These will go away after the 3rd or 4th day.

After the 7-day detox program, you can slowly re-introduce grains and dairy into your diet but you have to do these gradually. If you experience any symptoms when you consume any grain or dairy products, do not include them in your diet anymore as they may just cause more harm than good. It is still best to eat organic fruits and vegetable to lower the risk of consuming pesticides and insecticides usually found in commercial fruits and vegetables.

Undergoing a sugar detox can be overwhelming at first, but you will eventually make it. Just remember to follow the Tips For Staying On Track at Chapter 8 and the Natural Remedies For Sugar Cravings at Chapter 6.

Chapter 5: Foods To Avoid

To ensure that your blood sugar level stays normal, there are certain foods that you should not consume. Look at the list below:

Added sugars – During your detox, added sugars such as table sugar, corn syrup, beet, cane sugars, pancake syrup, maple syrup, malt syrup, molasses, liquid fructose, fructose sweetener, honey, fruit juice concentrate, crystal dextrose and anhydrous dextrose.

Alcohol – Alcoholic beverages can out a strain on your liver. During your detox, you need to stay away from any and all alcoholic drinks. This will give your liver a break and give it some time to heal properly.

Artificial sweeteners – Although advertised as better than sugar, studies show that artificial sweeteners such as Splenda, Equal and Aspartame causes toxicity in the liver. These artificial sweeteners are chemically manufactured products, and should be avoided at all costs; even after your detox.

Monosodium Glutamate (MSG) – This food additive is a common additive in Chinese foods. MSG, also known as glutamic acid, carrageenan, modified food starch or hydrolyzed vegetable protein. Monosodium Glutamate is an excitotoxin. Once consumed, it overexcites your cells, which can cause cell damage, or worse, even cell death. MSG is also in packaged foods so avoid consuming these products as well.

Coffee – Caffeine can cause a substantial rise in blood pressure. It can also cause the blood glucose level to go up. It is best to cut down your coffee intake gradually until you are down to one cup a day only. You may also switch to decaffeinated coffee until you are able to wean off completely.

Dairy Products – Even if you are not suffering from lactose intolerance, all dairy products are restricted during your detox because digesting such products puts a heavy strain on your detoxification system.

Packaged foods – All packaged foods are restricted during your detox. These products are heavily processed and laced with preservatives that are bad for your health.

Red Meat – Consuming too much red meat can put a strain on your liver, causing toxins to build up in your system due to inflammation. Eliminating red meat will allow your body to flush out toxins efficiently during your detox.

Unhealthy fats – Any product that contains hydrogenated fats are off limits during your detox. Also not allowed are corn oil, soy oil and any refined cooking oils.

Processed carbohydrates – Carbohydrates are broken down to sugar and are stored by the body as fats when consumed in large amounts. All flour products such as breads, pastas, pastries, etc should be avoided.

Chapter 6: Natural Remedies To Cure Sugar Cravings

Sugar stimulates dopamine in the brain, the same receptor that heroine stimulates. This is the reason sugar addicts are unable to control their urge to consume sugary products most of the time. If you are unable to control your sugar cravings, try these natural remedies.

1. Make sure that you consume enough protein for breakfast and have smaller meals throughout your day. Do not consume red meat as it can cause inflammation in the liver. Add fruits to each meal to curb down your cravings for dessert. Experts advise to consume sweet snacks with protein to keep blood sugar levels stable and prevent future cravings.

2. Chew some leaves of Gymnema Sylvestre or sprinkle a few powdered Gymnema on your tongue to suppress your appetite for sweets. This herb came from India, and it makes sweet goods less satisfying. For instance, fruit juice tastes like water after munching on Gymnema leaves. The effect will last for 15 minutes. This is enough time for you to control your craving.

3. Ginseng – Experts consider ginseng as a potential treatment for blood sugar levels. Consuming Ginseng helps reduce overeating and stress without affecting your mood, energy level or appetite.

4. Fenugreek – This herb has a mild sweet taste and smells like maple syrup. If you feel the urge to eat sugar-laced foods, chew on some fenugreek leaves or seeds. This herb also helps prevent spikes in blood sugar levels.

With the help of these natural remedies, it will be easier for you to cut down your sugar consumption. Sometimes, knowing that you can do something to control your urge for eating sweets gives you confidence and enables you to control your cravings successfully.

Furthermore, these remedies are all natural, so they do not have any harmful effects in the body. As long as the remedy you are using comes from natural sources and not from a Chemist's lab, you should be okay.

Chapter 7: Kick Sugar And Lose Weight

Eating fat does not make you gain weight. Its sugar and carbohydrates that makes you fat. Sugar raises insulin in the body. Insulin promotes fat storage. Therefore, when you consume foods rich in sugar, your body stores more fats, leading to faster weight gain.

Sugar addiction causes depression. Furthermore, when you consume too much sugar, your body stores it as fats instead of energy, making you feel weak and exhausted. Sugar also affects insulin level in your body that can lead to diabetes.

Sugar detox means to correct your blood sugar. After the detox, you will notice that your energy is higher, your sugar cravings are out and you have better skin. As a rule, it is best to eat whole, organic fruits and vegetables and grass-fed animals.

Kicking sugar out of your system may not be easy for the first few days. However, the result certainly overcomes any hardships you may encounter. Not only will you have a healthier body, you will also experience better sleep, less bloating, better mood and more consistent energy. Most of the people who already underwent the Sugar detox program claim that they no longer want to go back to their old habits and they are able to resist their yearning for sweet treats better.

Chapter 8: Tips For Staying On Track

Quitting any type of addiction is not easy. Here are some helpful tips to help you get through your sugar detox diet effectively.

- Do not skip meals. This is very important. Make sure you have enough fruits, vegetables and protein especially for breakfast. Eat in smaller portions when you are hungry, especially for snacks. Fruits and nuts are highly recommended.

- Always brings healthy snacks with you. Since you are cutting carbohydrates rich and sugary foods from your diet, you may feel hungry often. When you are hungry, your tendency to crave for food is increased. Again, fruits and nuts are the best for satisfying your hunger.

- To ensure that you do not skip meals and you always have some healthy snacks with you, stock your home with healthy foods. Also, prepare your meals ahead of time. During weekends, plan your meals for the weekdays and store them in the fridge. You can double a recipe that will last for a few days or cut your vegetables and store them in a container so that cooking is much easier.

- Check the labels for hidden sugars. Most food products contain added sugar. Although some products contain just a little bit of added sugars, it can still aggravate your cravings so watch what you buy.

- Create healthier habits. When you feel the urge to slip back to your old habits, remind yourself why you are doing this and focus on the thought that you are making a positive change. If you feel like having some sweet dessert after lunch, have some fruits. Do you feel like munching on something while reading your favorite book? Prepare some lightly salted popcorn for your snack. When the urge to cheat hits you, find ways to counter it.

- Drink enough water. Water helps flush out toxins from the body. Drinking water also helps alleviate some withdrawal symptoms during your detox.

- Since this sugar detox is only for 7 days, it would be best to stay away from parties during the 7-day period. Consuming alcohol is restricted during detox and party foods are often rich in carbohydrates and sugar.

- Drink a glass of water with lemon first thing in the morning. This helps stimulate your liver and digestive system to flush out all the accumulated toxins in your body.

At the end of the day, your determination and focus is still the key to a successful sugar detox plan. Always remember the reason you are doing this and keep in mind the benefits that this detox plan offers you. Every time you see a positive effect, acknowledge it and use it to fuel your desire to keep going.

Chapter 9: 7 Day Sugar Detox Diet Plan

For this sugar detox diet plan, you will have 3 meals a day with 2 snacks in between. It is also best to stop eating anything 3 hours before you go to sleep.

DAY 1

Breakfast

- Spinach and Berries Smoothie

Lunch

- Roasted Lemon Chicken and some fruits.

Dinner

- Leftover roasted chicken with hearty salad

DAY 2

Breakfast

- Pitted Fruits Smoothie

Lunch

- Roasted salmon with stir-fried veggies. You may have berries for dessert.

Dinner

- Left-over stir-fried veggies with green salad

DAY 4

Breakfast

- Creamy Peach Spice Smoothie

Lunch

- Baked Tilapia with Mango – Jicama Salad

Dinner

- Roasted Herbed Lemon Shrimp

DAY 5

Breakfast

- Almond Berry Smoothie

Lunch

- Crock pot Chili Black Beans with Tomato Peach Salad

  You can store your leftovers and use them for your next meals.

Dinner

- Leftover Chili Black Beans and some berries

DAY 6

Breakfast

- Tropical Blueberry Smoothie

Lunch

- Roasted Shrimp with herbs and Corn Squash Salad

Dinner

- Tuna Lettuce Wraps

DAY 7

Breakfast

- Mango-Berry-Cashew Smoothie

Lunch

- Turkey Soup with Green Fruity salad

Dinner

- Leftover Turkey Soup

You can have 2 ounces chocolate (70% or more) for snacks in between only after the fourth day of your detox. If you have allergic reactions to any of the ingredients, do not attempt to consume. You can try another recipe that suits you.

For snacks in between meals, if you feel hungry, munch on nuts and fruits. If you feel a great urge to eat sweet goodies, use any of the natural ways to suppress cravings found on Chapter 6.

Chapter 10: Sugar Detox Smoothie Recipes

You will surely enjoy these deliciously satisfying smoothies that are approved for your Sugar Detox plan.

1. **Morning Boost Smoothie**

   8 ounces Water

   4 ounces Nuts

   ½ Avocado

   2 teaspoons Almond Butter (organic)

   2 tablespoons plant-based Protein Powder

   A pinch of Salt

   Stevia as sweetener

2. **Pitted Fruits Smoothie**

   4 Peaches

   1 Avocado

   12 Cherries

   Some Ice

   Almond Milk (for consistency)

   2 tablespoons plant-based Protein Powder

3. **Spinach and Berries Smoothie**

   1 cup Blueberries or Raspberries

1 cup Spinach

2 cups Coconut Milk

1 tablespoon unrefined Coconut Oil

2 tablespoons plant-based Protein Powder

4. Creamy Peach Spice Smoothie

1 cup Peaches (frozen)

2 cups Coconut Milk (whole fat)

2 teaspoon Pumpkin Pie Spice (you can mix cinnamon, allspice and nutmeg if you can't find one)

1 teaspoon Ginger, grated

2 tablespoons plant-based protein powder (Vanilla flavor)

Toasted/raw Coconut for toppings

5. Almond Berry Smoothie

1 cup Almonds

Almond milk (enough to cover nuts when placed in the blender)

5 to 10 drops Stevia extract (depending on your taste)

1 teaspoon Vanilla extract

3 cups frozen Berries (blackberry, raspberry or blueberry)

1 Apple

1 Pear

Coconut water (depending on the consistency you want)

2 tablespoons plant-based Protein Powder

6. Tropical Blueberry Smoothie

½ cup Almond Milk (unsweetened)

1 cup Blueberries

½ ripe Mango

½ cup Pineapple

1 tablespoon Spirulina

1 tablespoon raw Cacao Powder

1 tablespoon unrefined Coconut Oil

2 tablespoons plant-based Protein Powder (Vanilla flavor)

7. Mango-Berry-Cashew Smoothie

1 cup Cashews

1 cup Coconut Water

½ cup Blueberries

½ cup Blackberries

1 ripe Mango, diced

2 tablespoons plant-based Protein Powder (Vanilla powder)

8. Peppermint Cashew Smoothie

1 ½ cups Peppermint Tea (warm)

1 tablespoon Cacao powder

1 tablespoon Coconut Oil (melted)

2 tablespoon Cashew nuts

2 teaspoons Spirulina

½ teaspoon Stevia extract

A pinch of salt

9. Kale and Berry Smoothie

1 cup Coconut Water

1 cup mixed Berries (Raspberry, Strawberry and Cherry)

2 dates

1 cup Kale

2 tablespoons plant-based Protein Powder

1 tablespoon Flax Seeds (ground)

10. Choco Blueberry Smoothie

1 cup Blueberries (fresh or frozen)

½ cup Spinach

A dash of Cinnamon

1 tablespoon raw Cacao

2 tablespoons Almond Butter

½ cup Coconut Milk

½ cup Coconut Water

A dash of Stevia (according to your taste)

2 tablespoons plant-based Protein Powder

1 tablespoon Flax Seeds (ground)

These smoothie recipes fit perfectly in your Sugar Detox diet. After taking a glass of smoothie for breakfast, you may eat some berries and nuts. Eat only a handful of nuts per snack time and no more. You can consume as much berries and fruits as you want.

Conclusion

Thank you again for purchasing this book on **Sugar Detox!**

I am extremely excited to pass this information along to you, and I am so happy that you now have read and can hopefully implement these strategies going forward.

I hope this book was able to help you understand more about added sugar, and how to curb your sugar cravings for a stable blood sugar level and better health.

The next step is to get started using this information and to hopefully live a healthier, more energetic and happier life!

Please don't be someone who just reads this information and doesn't apply it, the strategies in this book will only benefit you if you use them!

If you know of anyone else that could benefit from the information presented here please inform them of this book.

Finally, if you enjoyed this book and feel it has added value to your life in any way, please take the time to share your thoughts and post a review on Amazon. It'd be greatly appreciated!

Thank you and good luck!

Preview Of:

Anti-Inflammatory Diet: The #1 Anti Inflammatory Recipe Guide!

<u>Anti-Inflammatory Diet</u>

Eliminate Pain, Heal Yourself, Combat Heart Disease, And Fight Inflammation Using Food!

Introduction

I want to thank you and congratulate you for purchasing the book, "Anti Inflammatory Diet: The #1 Anti-Inflammatory Recipe Guide! - Eliminate Pain, Heal Yourself, Combat Heart Disease and Fight Inflammation Using Food".

This "Anti Inflammatory Diet" book contains proven steps and strategies on how to fight inflammation through holistic approach.

Inflammation is the body's natural response to infection and injuries. It is essential to start the healing process. Redness, pain, swelling and heat are symptoms which mean that the body is triggering the immune system to fight foreign bodies and start tissue repair. The problem arises when the healthy cells are damaged in the aftermath of inflammation.

Inflammation is linked to major chronic illness like heart diseases, stroke and diabetes. Fortunately, people are not powerless in preventing inflammation from going out of control. By ensuring that you have a healthy lifestyle, you are relieving your body from toxins and prevent common chronic illness.

Adopting healthy habits can dramatically improve your inflammation symptoms. This is a combination of a healthy diet and good habits. Fuel your body with natural anti-inflammatory foods to keep your joints functioning well.

Take control of your life and start living a healthy lifestyle to feel better.

Thanks again for purchasing this book, I hope you enjoy it!

Chapter 1: Anti-inflammatory Diet Guidelines

Unlike other diets, the anti-inflammatory diet is different since it is solely focused on weight loss. It is more of a dietary guideline for life than a short term diet.

There are also more than one approach to the anti-inflammatory diet with each one having its own benefit. Many doctors say that the anti-inflammatory diet can benefit everyone and is good for overall health.

What is inflammation?

Inflammation is the body's response to harmful and irritating stimuli. It is the body's way of protecting itself by removing damaged cells, pathogens and irritants to encourage a faster healing process.

Inflammation is not the same as infection although infection can cause inflammation. Infection is caused by virus, fungus and bacteria while inflammation is the body's reaction to it.

Initially, inflammation is beneficial to your immune response. For example, if you cut yourself while cooking, you might notice the area swells and reddens. This response is essential in the healing process.

Types of inflammation

- Acute inflammation

Acute inflammation starts rapidly as soon as the injury is acquired. It can last for few minutes to only few days. The most common examples of acute inflammation are cuts, bruises and sore throat.

- Chronic inflammation

Chronic inflammation is long term and can even last for years. It usually results after the body has failed to eliminate the cause of acute inflammation. It is also a response to antigens. It happens when the body attacks healthy tissue because it mistakes it for harmful pathogens. Examples include asthma, tuberculosis and chronic sinusitis.

Signs of inflammation

- Pain. The inflicted area will be painful most especially when touched. Chemicals in the body are released in the nerve ending making the area much more sensitive.
- Redness. The redness happens because the capillaries are filled with more blood than usual.
- Immobility. Since the area is painful to touch, you might also experience loss of function.
- Swelling. This is caused by the accumulation of fluid in the affected area.
- Heat. More blood accumulates in the area which makes it warmer than the rest of the body.

What happens during inflammation?

You can feel the effect of inflammation immediately after the tissue is damaged. Acute inflammation occurs in three stages. First, the arterioles or the small branches of the arteries that supply blood to the different parts of the body dilate and results to an increase in blood flow. The capillaries become permeable and fluid and blood move in-between the spaces of cells. Neutrophilis which is a type of white blood cell that contains enzyme that digest microorganisms move out of the capillaries. It then transfers to the spaces between the cells.

The Neutrophilis is the body's first line of defense since it contains enzymes that can destroy bacteria and prevent infections. However, it also contains inflammatory properties which can lead to heart ailments and autoimmune disease.

Function of the anti-inflammatory diet

Physicians and medical experts may recommend anti-inflammatory diets to lessen the effect of inflammation in the body. The diet is usually prescribed with other medicines but you can also follow it to simply reduce inflammation symptoms in your system. Adding foods that improve symptoms of chronic disease supplies the body with the needed nutrients to decrease body inflammation.

Thanks for Previewing My Exciting Book Entitled:

"Anti-Inflammatory Diet: The #1 Anti Inflammatory Recipe Guide! Eliminate Pain, Heal Yourself, Combat Heart Disease, And Fight Inflammation Using Food!"

To purchase this book, simply go to the Amazon Kindle store and simply search:

"ANTI-INFLAMMATORY DIET"

Then just scroll down until you see my book. You will know it is mine because you will see my name "Sarah Brooks" underneath the title.

Alternatively, you can visit my author page on Amazon to see this book and other work I have done. Thanks so much, and please don't forget your free bonuses

DON'T LEAVE YET! - CHECK OUT YOUR FREE BONUSES BELOW!

Free Bonus Offer: Get Free Access To The www.LiveFitVIP.com VIP Newsletter!

Once you enter your email address you will immediately get free access to this awesome newsletter!

But wait, right now if you join now for free you will also get free access to the "The 7 Keys To Body Transformation" free EBook!

To claim both your FREE VIP NEWSLETTER MEMBERSHIP and your FREE BONUS EBook on THE 7 KEYS TO BODY TRANSFORMATION!

Just Go To:

www.liveFitVIP.com